STRUCTURAL INTEGRATION EXPLAINED

A Comprehensive Guide To Myofascial Release, Body Alignment, Postural Correction, And Holistic Healing Techniques

DR. MELISSA STOTLER

Disclaimer:

The data in this book, is solely meant to be informative and instructional.

This book is not intended to replace expert medical advice, diagnosis, or care. No medical, health, or other professional services are offered by the author, publisher, or any affiliated parties

Individual outcomes may differ in the practice of these therapies, which entail a variety of approaches and methodologies.

A one-on-one session with a trained or certified healthcare professional is still preferable. It is best to consult a trained healthcare provider before making any decisions regarding your health.

The author of this book is not affiliated with any specific website, product, or organization related to any of these therapies.

All reasonable measures have been taken by the author and publisher to guarantee the authenticity and dependability of the material contained in this book.

Contents

ABOUT THIS BOOK

The book Structural Integration Explained serves as an essential guide for anyone looking to understand and benefit from this transformative approach to bodywork. It begins by delving into the foundational elements of human anatomy, offering readers a comprehensive overview of the fascial system, muscles, and joints while explaining common misalignments that Structural Integration is designed to address. This foundational knowledge is crucial for grasping how Structural Integration can enhance body alignment and movement efficiency.

The book then explores the core principles of Structural Integration, including the widely recognized ten-series approach. Readers will gain insight into how this structured protocol systematically addresses body alignment, posture, and movement patterns. Techniques for releasing tension and integrating body systems are explained, illustrating how Structural Integration promotes overall physical harmony.

A key section of the book is dedicated to the practitioner's role, highlighting the rigorous training and certification required to practice effectively. It provides a detailed look at what clients can expect during sessions, the importance of clear communication between practitioner and client, and the ethical standards that guide professional practice. Additionally, it emphasizes the necessity of continuous education to maintain and enhance one's skills.

For those preparing for their first session, the book offers practical advice on what to expect during the initial consultation, how to prepare, and what to communicate to ensure a successful experience. It also covers post-session care to help clients maximize the benefits of their sessions.

Techniques and methods are thoroughly examined, including deep tissue work, myofascial release, and specific Rolfing techniques. Self-care practices are also discussed, empowering readers to continue benefiting from Structural Integration outside of their sessions.

The book addresses common conditions that Structural Integration can effectively treat, such as chronic pain, postural imbalances, and sports injuries. It also outlines strategies for integrating these practices into daily life, from daily routines and ergonomics to stress management and lifestyle adjustments.

To assist in evaluating progress, readers are guided on how to track improvements, provide feedback, and maintain results over time. Tools for self-assessment and periodic reviews are included to support ongoing development and success.

The book answers common concerns and FAQs, including safety, cost, finding a practitioner, and understanding session frequency. It provides clear and practical information to help readers make informed decisions and achieve long-term benefits from Structural Integration.

CHAPTER ONE

UNDERSTANDING THE ANATOMY

Basic Anatomy Overview

Structural Integration (SI) relies on a solid understanding of human anatomy to effectively address and improve the body's alignment and function. At its core, human anatomy is about how different parts of the body are organized and how they work together.

The human body is divided into several systems, including the skeletal system, muscular system, and fascial system. The skeletal system provides the body's framework, consisting of bones and joints that support and protect internal organs. The muscular system comprises muscles that enable movement and stability. The fascial system is a connective tissue network that envelops and supports muscles, organs, and other structures, playing a crucial role in maintaining body integrity and function.

In Structural Integration, understanding these systems is vital because SI works to align and balance the body's structure. By addressing imbalances and restrictions within these systems, SI practitioners aim to enhance overall body function and alleviate discomfort.

Fascial System

The fascial system is an extensive network of connective tissues that permeates the entire body. It includes the fascia, a thin yet strong tissue that wraps around muscles, bones, and organs, binding them together and allowing them to move smoothly against one another.

Fascia comes in different forms, including superficial fascia (which lies just under the skin), deep fascia (which surrounds muscles and separates them into compartments), and visceral fascia (which envelops organs). The health and flexibility of the fascia are critical for optimal body movement and alignment. When fascia becomes restricted or bound, it can lead to pain, reduced mobility, and poor posture.

Structural Integration aims to release these fascial restrictions through targeted techniques, allowing the body to return to its natural alignment and function. By working with the fascial system, SI practitioners help restore balance and ease to the entire body.

Muscles And Joints

Muscles and joints are integral comMponents of the body's movement system, and their interaction with the fascia is essential for functional movement. Muscles are responsible for generating force and facilitating movement by contracting and relaxing. Joints, where two or more bones meet, allow for various types of movement, including flexion, extension, and rotation.

The fascia wraps around muscles and joints, providing support and flexibility. This connective tissue helps to distribute forces generated by muscle contractions and stabilize joints during movement. When muscles and joints are not properly aligned or if fascia becomes restricted, it can disrupt this balance, leading to inefficiencies in movement and potential pain or injury.

Structural Integration addresses these issues by working to release tension in the fascia and realign the muscles and joints. This holistic approach helps restore proper movement patterns and reduce strain on the body's structures.

Common Misalignments

Structural Integration is designed to address several common misalignments and issues that affect body function and posture. One common misalignment is the forward head posture, where the head protrudes forward from the shoulders, often due to poor posture or prolonged sitting. This can lead to neck and back pain and reduced mobility.

Another issue is pelvic tilt, where the pelvis tilts excessively forward or backward, affecting spinal alignment and potentially causing lower back pain. Misalignments in the shoulders and hips can also occur, leading to uneven weight distribution and compensatory movements that can cause discomfort or injury.

SI aims to identify and correct these misalignments through a series of manual techniques and postural exercises. By addressing these issues, practitioners help improve overall alignment and reduce associated discomfort.

Anatomical Terminology

Understanding anatomical terminology is crucial for anyone involved in Structural Integration. Key terms include:

Anatomy: The study of the structure of the body and its parts.

Fascia: Connective tissue that surrounds muscles, organs, and other structures.

Muscle: Tissue capable of contracting to move.

Joint: The connection between two or more bones, allowing movement.

Posture: The alignment of the body in space.

Alignment: The arrangement of body parts about each other.

Familiarity with these terms helps practitioners communicate effectively and understand the specific areas they are working to address.

By grasping the terminology, practitioners can better follow and implement techniques to improve body function and alignment.

By comprehending these basic concepts, individuals involved in Structural Integration can gain a clearer understanding of the body's structure and function, leading to more effective and targeted treatment.

CHAPTER TWO

PRINCIPLES OF STRUCTURAL INTEGRATION

Structural Integration is based on the principle that the body is a unified whole, where the structure of one part affects the entire system. The main goal is to address and correct misalignments and imbalances in the body's connective tissues, primarily fascia, which encase and support muscles and organs.

The approach is founded on the belief that these misalignments can lead to chronic pain, reduced mobility, and inefficient movement patterns. By focusing on realigning and balancing the body's structure, Structural Integration aims to improve overall function and well-being.

The practice involves a series of manual therapies designed to lengthen and reshape the fascia. This process helps to release tension and restore proper alignment. By addressing the body's structural issues, it is believed that the body can achieve a more natural and efficient state, enhancing both physical performance and comfort.

The Ten-Series Approach: Explanation Of The Ten-Session Protocol

The Ten-Series is a core component of Structural Integration, consisting of a sequence of ten sessions, each designed to address different aspects of the body's structure. This protocol follows a systematic approach to improve overall alignment and function.

Sessions 1-3: The Superficial Fascia

These initial sessions focus on the superficial layers of fascia and aim to establish a foundation of balance. The work typically involves the upper body, including the chest, shoulders, and arms. The goal is to create a base for deeper work by improving the initial layers of tissue and alignment.

Sessions 4-7: The Core Fascia

The next set of sessions delves into the core fascia, including the abdominal and lower back regions. This phase targets the deeper layers of connective tissue, working to address issues in the core structure of the body. The focus is on integrating the upper and lower body, enhancing core stability and function.

Sessions 8-10: The Integration Phase

The final sessions aim to integrate the work done in the previous stages. This phase often includes addressing any remaining issues and refining the overall alignment and movement patterns. The goal is to ensure that the body functions as a cohesive unit, with improved balance and mobility.

Body Alignment And Posture: How Structural Integration Aims To Improve Alignment

One of the primary objectives of Structural Integration is to enhance body alignment and posture. Misalignment and poor posture can lead to various issues, including discomfort, pain, and reduced mobility. Structural Integration works by addressing these issues through targeted manipulation of the fascia.

The process involves assessing and correcting the alignment of the body's segments, including the spine, pelvis, and shoulders. By applying specific techniques to the connective tissues, practitioners help to release tension and realign the body's structure. This realignment can lead to improved posture, reducing strain on muscles and joints, and promoting a more balanced and natural stance.

Movement Patterns: The Impact Of Structural Integration On Movement Efficiency

Structural Integration also focuses on improving movement patterns and efficiency. Many people develop inefficient movement habits due to structural imbalances and restrictions in the body. These inefficient patterns can contribute to discomfort and reduce overall physical performance.

Through the Ten-Series approach, Structural Integration helps to identify and address these inefficient movement patterns. By improving the alignment and function of the body's structure, the technique aims to enhance movement efficiency. This can result in smoother, more fluid motions and better overall physical performance.

Release Techniques: Methods Used To Release Tension And Restrictions

Release techniques are central to Structural Integration. These methods are designed to alleviate tension and restrictions in the fascia, which can contribute to discomfort and dysfunction. Several techniques may be used during sessions, including:

Deep Tissue Manipulation: This involves applying pressure to specific areas of the fascia to release deep-seated tension and restrictions.

Myofascial Release: A technique that targets the myofascial tissue to improve flexibility and reduce pain by gently stretching and releasing the connective tissue.

Rolfing Techniques: A specialized method within Structural Integration that focuses on realigning the body's structure and improving overall posture and function.

These techniques work together to address various issues in the fascia, helping to restore balance and function to the body.

Integration Of Systems: How Different Systems In The Body Are Integrated

Structural Integration emphasizes the integration of different systems within the body to achieve overall balance and efficiency. This holistic approach involves aligning and coordinating the musculoskeletal, nervous, and connective tissue systems.

By addressing the connections between these systems, Structural Integration helps to create a more cohesive and functional body.

For example, improving alignment and reducing restrictions in the fascia can have a positive impact on the nervous system, enhancing overall bodily function and movement. The goal is to achieve a seamless integration of these systems, leading to improved posture, movement efficiency, and overall well-being.

CHAPTER THREE

THE PRACTITIONER'S ROLE

Training And Certification: Requirements And Qualifications For Practitioners

A structural integration practitioner plays a crucial role in helping clients achieve improved body alignment and function. To become a certified practitioner, one must complete extensive training in structural integration techniques and bodywork.

This training typically includes coursework in anatomy, physiology, and the principles of structural integration, combined with hands-on practice under the supervision of experienced instructors. Certification programs often require a significant number of hours of training and practical experience, ensuring that practitioners are well-equipped to assess and address client's needs effectively.

In addition to formal education, practitioners may also need to meet specific state or national certification requirements. These may include passing written and practical exams to demonstrate proficiency in the techniques and knowledge necessary for effective practice. Ongoing certification may also involve regular continuing education to stay current with advances in the field and maintain professional standards.

Session Structure: What A Typical Session Entails

A typical structural integration session is carefully structured to maximize the benefits for the client. The session generally begins with an assessment where the practitioner evaluates the client's posture, movement patterns, and any areas of tension or discomfort. This assessment helps in developing a customized treatment plan that targets specific areas of concern.

During the session, the practitioner applies a variety of hands-on techniques aimed at releasing tension, improving alignment, and enhancing overall body function. These techniques often involve deep tissue manipulation, myofascial release, and other methods designed to address the connective tissue and improve the body's structural balance. Sessions are usually conducted in a private, comfortable setting to ensure that the client can relax and fully engage in the process.

The session concludes with a review of the client's progress and any recommendations for follow-up treatments or self-care practices. The practitioner may also guide exercises or stretches to support the work done during the session and promote long-term benefits.

Client Communication: Importance of Understanding Client Needs and Goals

Effective communication between the practitioner and the client is essential for a successful structural integration experience. At the outset, the practitioner should conduct a thorough consultation to understand the client's specific needs, goals, and any medical history or concerns that may impact the treatment.

This dialogue helps in tailoring the session to address the client's unique situation and ensures that their expectations are realistic and achievable.

Throughout the treatment process, ongoing communication is crucial. The practitioner should regularly check in with the client to gauge their comfort level, discuss any changes in their condition, and adjust the treatment plan as necessary.

Encouraging open and honest feedback allows the practitioner to make informed adjustments and ensures that the client feels heard and valued.

Ethics And Professionalism: Maintaining Professionalism In Practice

Maintaining high ethical standards and professionalism is fundamental in structural integration practice.

Practitioners are expected to adhere to a code of ethics that prioritizes client safety, respect, and confidentiality. This includes obtaining informed consent before beginning any treatment, being transparent about the techniques used, and respecting the client's boundaries.

Professionalism also extends to maintaining appropriate boundaries and conducting oneself in a manner that fosters trust and respect. Practitioners should be punctual, reliable, and dedicated to providing the highest standard of care. This professionalism not only enhances the client's experience but also upholds the integrity of the practice.

Continuous Education: The Need For Ongoing Learning And Development

The field of structural integration is continually evolving, with new research, techniques, and advancements emerging regularly.

To provide the best possible care, practitioners must engage in continuous education and professional development.

This may involve attending workshops, conferences, and advanced training programs to stay updated on the latest developments in the field.

Ongoing learning helps practitioners refine their skills, broaden their knowledge base, and incorporate new techniques into their practice. It also supports their ability to address a wide range of client needs and adapt to changes in the field.

Committing to lifelong learning ensures that practitioners remain at the forefront of their profession and continue to offer effective, evidence-based care.

CHAPTER FOUR

PREPARING FOR YOUR FIRST SESSION

Initial Consultation: What To Expect During The First Meeting

The initial consultation for Structural Integration is your opportunity to meet your practitioner and discuss your personal goals and concerns. During this meeting, the practitioner will ask you about your medical history, any previous injuries, and current issues you're facing. They will want to understand your daily activities, lifestyle, and any specific goals you have in mind for the treatment. This conversation helps them tailor the sessions to fit your needs precisely.

You'll likely be asked about your physical habits, such as how often you exercise or if you have any posture-related issues. The practitioner will also explain the Structural Integration process, including what techniques they will use and how these can benefit you. This is the time to ask any questions you have about the treatment, so don't hesitate to voice your concerns or curiosities. The goal is to ensure that you feel comfortable and informed before beginning the actual sessions.

Assessment And Goals: How The Practitioner Assesses Your Needs

Assessment is a crucial part of Structural Integration. Your practitioner will start by evaluating your posture, movement patterns, and the alignment of your body. They may use various techniques such as visual inspection, palpation, or even functional tests to identify areas of tension or imbalance.

The practitioner will discuss your assessment findings with you, explaining how they plan to address any issues. They will also help you set realistic goals for your treatment. These goals could range from improving flexibility and reducing pain to enhancing overall body alignment and posture. By understanding your specific needs and goals, the practitioner can create a customized treatment plan that addresses the root causes of your discomfort and supports your desired outcomes.

Session Preparation: How To Prepare For A Session

Preparing for a Structural Integration session involves a few simple but important steps. First, wear comfortable, loose-fitting clothing that allows for easy movement. The sessions typically require you to be partially or fully unclothed, so it's helpful to bring or wear appropriate clothing such as shorts and a tank top. Make sure to discuss clothing preferences with your practitioner beforehand to ensure you are comfortable.

It's also beneficial to arrive at your session hydrated and to avoid eating a heavy meal right before. Your practitioner may advise you to refrain from vigorous exercise or strenuous activities on the day of your session. Arriving a bit early can give you time to relax and mentally prepare, making the session more effective and enjoyable.

What To Communicate: Information To Share With Your Practitioner

Clear communication with your practitioner is essential for a successful Structural Integration experience. Share any physical discomfort or areas of pain you are experiencing, as well as any changes in your condition since your last session. Inform them about any new injuries or health issues that could impact your treatment.

Be open about your feelings and reactions during the session. If something feels uncomfortable or painful, let your practitioner know immediately. This feedback is crucial for adjusting the techniques and ensuring that the treatment is effective and comfortable for you. Additionally, communicate any specific goals or changes you wish to see, so the practitioner can tailor the sessions to your evolving needs.

Post-Session Care: Steps To Take After Your First Session

After your first Structural Integration session, it's important to follow a few post-session care steps to maximize the benefits and support your body's adjustment. Hydrate well to help flush out toxins and reduce muscle soreness.

Drinking plenty of water can aid in the healing process and keep your body well-hydrated.

Rest and avoid any strenuous activities for the remainder of the day. Gentle stretching or light movement may help ease any initial discomfort. If you experience soreness, applying a warm compress or taking a warm bath can be soothing. Pay attention to how your body responds to the session, and communicate any significant reactions or concerns to your practitioner.

Finally, maintain the recommended follow-up schedule and adhere to any additional instructions given by your practitioner. These steps are essential for achieving the best results from your Structural Integration treatment and for supporting your body's overall alignment and well-being.

CHAPTER FIVE

TECHNIQUES AND METHODS

Basic Techniques: Common Techniques Used In Structural Integration

Structural Integration employs a variety of techniques designed to balance the body's structure and improve overall function. One fundamental technique involves postural assessment and body mapping, where practitioners evaluate your posture and alignment to identify areas of imbalance. Following this, manual therapy techniques are applied to address these imbalances.

Deep tissue manipulation is another basic technique, that focuses on the deeper layers of muscles and connective tissues. The goal here is to release chronic tension and improve circulation. This often involves using slow, deliberate strokes to apply pressure to the targeted areas.

Movement re-education is also a crucial part of the process. This technique involves guiding you through specific movements to enhance body awareness and facilitate better movement patterns. By integrating these techniques, Structural Integration aims to create a more balanced and efficient body structure.

Deep Tissue Work: Focus On Deep Fascial Layers

Deep tissue work in Structural Integration targets the deeper layers of fascia and muscle tissue to address chronic tension and dysfunction. The fascia is a connective tissue that surrounds muscles and organs, and when it becomes tight or restricted, it can lead to pain and limited movement.

Applying sustained pressure is a core method used in deep tissue work. This involves using the fingers, thumbs, or elbows to apply firm pressure to the affected areas, gradually working through the layers of tissue to release adhesions and improve flexibility.

Cross-fiber friction is another technique used to break down scar tissue and adhesions within the fascia. By applying pressure perpendicular to the direction of the fibers, this method helps to realign and smooth the tissue, promoting better movement and function.

In deep tissue work, the practitioner may also incorporate stretching and joint mobilization techniques to enhance the overall effect. These methods help to improve the range of motion and support the body's natural healing processes.

Myofascial Release: Methods For Releasing Tightness In The Fascia

Myofascial release focuses on relieving tightness and restrictions within the fascia, the connective tissue that encases muscles and organs. This technique is crucial for addressing areas of chronic tension and improving overall movement.

Gentle, sustained pressure is applied to areas of tightness to help release fascial restrictions. The practitioner uses their hands to apply gentle, consistent pressure, allowing the fascia to gradually release and stretch.

Active release techniques involve guiding the client through specific movements while applying pressure to the affected fascia. This helps to break up adhesions and improve the elasticity of the fascia.

Myofascial stretching is another important method where the practitioner applies a gentle stretch to the fascia, aiming to increase flexibility and reduce tension. This technique often involves holding the stretch for a few minutes to allow the fascia to adapt and release.

Overall, myofascial release methods are designed to address and alleviate chronic tightness, improve range of motion, and enhance overall body function.

Rolfing Techniques: Specific Techniques Related to Rolfing, a Form of Structural Integration

Rolfing is a specific form of Structural Integration that employs a variety of techniques to reorganize the body's connective tissue and improve alignment. Developed by

Ida Rolf, Rolfing focuses on achieving structural balance and enhancing functional movement.

The Rolfing Ten Series is a well-known approach within Rolfing, consisting of ten sessions that progressively address different aspects of the body.

Each session targets specific areas, starting with the superficial layers and gradually moving deeper to address more complex issues.

Deep connective tissue manipulation is a key Rolfing technique, where the practitioner uses their hands, elbows, or forearms to apply deep pressure to the connective tissue. This technique aims to release restrictions and promote better alignment.

Structural re-education involves guiding the client through specific movements and postural adjustments to reinforce the changes achieved during the sessions. This helps to ensure that the body maintains a new, more balanced alignment over time.

Rolfing techniques are designed to create lasting changes in the body's structure, improve movement patterns, and enhance overall well-being.

Self-Care Practices: Techniques You Can Use Between Sessions

Self-care practices are essential for maintaining the benefits of Structural Integration and promoting ongoing body health. Here are some techniques you can use between sessions:

Foam rolling is a self-myofascial release technique that helps to relieve muscle tightness and improve circulation.

By rolling a foam roller over specific areas, you can apply gentle pressure to the fascia and muscles, helping to release tension and increase flexibility.

Stretching exercises are crucial for maintaining flexibility and reducing muscle tightness. Incorporate a routine of dynamic and static stretches to target major muscle groups and fascia throughout your body.

Mindful movement practices, such as yoga or tai chi, can help improve body awareness and support the alignment changes achieved in Structural Integration.

These practices promote balance, flexibility, and relaxation, contributing to overall body health.

Hydration and nutrition play a significant role in maintaining the health of your connective tissues. Drink plenty of water and eat a balanced diet rich in nutrients to support tissue repair and overall well-being.

By integrating these self-care practices into your routine, you can enhance the results of your Structural Integration sessions and support long-term health and well-being.

CHAPTER SIX

COMMON CONDITIONS ADDRESSED

Chronic Pain: How Structural Integration Can Help With Chronic Pain Conditions

Structural Integration offers a comprehensive approach to managing chronic pain. Chronic pain often stems from unresolved musculoskeletal issues, including misalignments and muscle imbalances. Structural Integration works by realigning the body and releasing restrictions in the connective tissue.

During a Structural Integration session, a practitioner assesses and manipulates the fascia, the connective tissue surrounding muscles, bones, and organs. By focusing on these areas, the treatment aims to reduce pain by addressing the root causes rather than just masking symptoms. For individuals with chronic pain, such as those suffering from lower back pain or neck tension, Structural Integration helps improve alignment and restore functional movement, which can significantly alleviate discomfort and enhance quality of life.

Postural Imbalances: Addressing Issues Related To Poor Posture

Postural imbalances are often a result of prolonged poor posture, such as sitting at a desk for long periods or slouching. These imbalances can lead to discomfort, pain, and even long-term health issues. Structural Integration targets these issues by focusing on the body's alignment and movement patterns.

Through a series of sessions, the practitioner evaluates the client's posture and identifies areas where the body is compensating for misalignments. Techniques used during Structural Integration work to lengthen and align the fascia, which helps to correct postural imbalances. As a result, clients experience improved posture, reduced muscle tension, and a more balanced and efficient movement pattern. This process not only enhances overall posture but also reduces the risk of future postural-related problems.

Sports Injuries: Benefits For Athletes And Injury Recovery

For athletes, Structural Integration provides valuable benefits in both injury recovery and performance enhancement. Sports injuries often result in muscle strains, joint issues, and imbalances caused by repetitive movements or trauma. Structural Integration addresses these concerns by focusing on the body's connective tissues and alignment.

The treatment helps by promoting efficient movement patterns and facilitating the body's natural healing processes. Techniques are tailored to release tension, correct imbalances, and enhance flexibility. This targeted approach helps athletes recover more swiftly from injuries, reduces the risk of future injuries, and improves overall performance. Whether recovering from a sprain or striving to enhance mobility and strength, Structural Integration offers a supportive role in the athlete's recovery and conditioning process.

Stress And Tension: Managing Stress And Muscular Tension

Structural Integration can be an effective method for managing stress and reducing muscular tension. Chronic stress often manifests physically as muscle tightness, especially in areas like the shoulders, neck, and back. By addressing the body's connective tissue and realigning the structure, Structural Integration helps to alleviate these physical manifestations of stress.

Sessions involve deep tissue work and stretching, which not only releases muscular tension but also promotes relaxation and a sense of well-being. As the fascia is worked on and realigned, clients often experience a decrease in overall tension, improved mood, and better stress management. Regular Structural Integration sessions can be a valuable part of a holistic approach to managing stress and maintaining physical and emotional balance.

Rehabilitation Support: Supporting Recovery from Various Physical Conditions

Structural Integration is also beneficial in supporting recovery from various physical conditions. Whether recovering from surgery, injury, or chronic conditions like arthritis, this therapy helps facilitate the body's healing process. By focusing on the connective tissue, Structural Integration assists in improving movement patterns, reducing pain, and restoring functionality.

During rehabilitation, Structural Integration practitioners work to release restrictions in the fascia and improve overall body alignment. This approach supports better movement mechanics and reduces compensatory patterns that could impede recovery. For individuals undergoing rehabilitation, this therapy offers a complementary method to traditional treatments, enhancing overall recovery and aiding in the restoration of normal function.

CHAPTER SEVEN

INTEGRATING STRUCTURAL INTEGRATION INTO DAILY LIFE

Integrating Structural Integration into daily life involves applying the principles and practices learned during your sessions to your everyday activities.

This approach ensures that the benefits you gain from Structural Integration continue to enhance your well-being long after your sessions have ended.

Daily Practices: How To Incorporate Principles Into Your Daily Routine

One effective way to incorporate Structural Integration principles into your daily routine is to focus on body awareness and alignment. Start by regularly checking in with your posture—are you standing tall with your shoulders relaxed? Practice gentle body scans where you mentally assess areas of tension or discomfort. Integrate these checks into your daily activities, such as while working at your desk or standing in line.

Additionally, use mindful breathing exercises to promote relaxation and awareness. Deep, diaphragmatic breathing can help release tension and improve your overall body awareness.

Incorporating these practices into your routine can create a lasting impact on your body's alignment and comfort.

Exercise And Movement: Complementary Exercises To Support Structural Integration

Complementary exercises are crucial for reinforcing the benefits of Structural

Integration. Focus on movements that enhance flexibility, strength, and body awareness. Stretching exercises, such as yoga or Pilates, can help maintain the length and suppleness of your muscles and connective tissues, supporting the structural changes achieved during your sessions.

Strength-building exercises should emphasize core stability and balance. Core exercises, like planks and bridges, help support your spine and improve overall body alignment.

Integrate these exercises into your weekly routine to keep your body strong and well-aligned.

Incorporate regular movement into your day, whether through walking, swimming, or cycling.

Consistent, varied physical activity helps maintain the benefits of Structural Integration and keeps your body in optimal condition.

Ergonomics: Improving Posture And Body Mechanics At Work

Improving ergonomics at your workplace is essential for maintaining good posture and preventing strain.

Begin by adjusting your workstation to ensure that your desk, chair, and computer screen are set at the correct heights. Your chair should support your lower back, and your feet should rest flat on the floor.

Practice proper body mechanics when sitting or standing. Avoid slouching by sitting back in your chair and keeping your shoulders relaxed. When standing, distribute your weight evenly between both feet.

If you spend long hours at your desk, take regular breaks to stretch and move around to prevent stiffness and discomfort.

Stress Management: Techniques To Manage Stress And Maintain Results

Stress can impact your body's alignment and overall well-being. Implement stress management techniques to help maintain the benefits of Structural Integration.

Mindfulness and meditation practices are excellent for reducing stress and enhancing body awareness. Spend a few minutes each day in quiet reflection, focusing on your breath and relaxation.

In addition, physical activities such as yoga or tai chi can help manage stress by combining gentle movement with mindful breathing. Regular exercise also plays a significant role in stress reduction. Find activities that you enjoy and make time for them regularly.

Lifestyle Adjustments: Small Changes for Overall Well-Being

Small lifestyle adjustments can significantly impact your overall well-being.

Start by incorporating healthy eating habits, focusing on a balanced diet rich in nutrients that support muscle and joint health. Hydration is also crucial; drink plenty of water to keep your tissues well-hydrated.

Ensure that you get adequate sleep each night, as quality rest is vital for your body's recovery and maintenance.

Develop a consistent sleep routine to support restful sleep. Lastly, cultivate positive habits such as regular social interaction and engaging in hobbies to enhance your mental and emotional well-being.

By making these practical adjustments, you can seamlessly integrate the principles of Structural Integration into your daily life, supporting long-term health and alignment.

CHAPTER EIGHT

EVALUATING PROGRESS

Evaluating progress in Structural Integration is essential to ensure that the treatment is effective and that you are moving toward your desired outcomes.

This process involves a combination of objective measurements and subjective feedback to gauge how well the treatment is working.

To start, it's important to track various indicators of improvement, such as changes in posture, flexibility, and pain levels.

These indicators can be assessed through regular physical evaluations and measurements taken at different stages of the treatment.

For instance, you might notice an increased range of motion or reduced discomfort in areas that were previously problematic.

Keeping detailed records of these changes will help you and your practitioner determine the effectiveness of the treatment.

Additionally, improvements can be measured through functional assessments. These assessments evaluate how well you can perform daily activities and tasks that were previously difficult.

This can include simple tasks like walking or more complex movements related to your specific goals.

By comparing these functional assessments over time, you can better understand the progress you've made and identify any areas that might need further attention.

Tracking Improvements: How to Measure Progress and Outcomes

Tracking improvements involves systematically documenting changes and outcomes to understand how well the treatment is working. One effective method is to use standardized questionnaires or scales that measure pain levels, functional ability, and quality of life. These tools provide a quantifiable way to assess progress and can help in identifying trends over time.

Another practical approach is to take regular photos or videos of your posture and movement patterns.

Comparing these visual records can provide a clear indication of how your body is changing in response to treatment.

Ensure that the photos or videos are taken under similar conditions each time to maintain consistency.

Furthermore, maintaining a journal where you note daily experiences, improvements, and any challenges encountered can be invaluable. This personal record can help in understanding subtle changes that may not be immediately noticeable but contribute to overall progress.

Feedback And Adjustments: Providing Feedback To Your Practitioner And Adjusting Goals

Providing feedback to your practitioner is a crucial part of the treatment process. Regularly discussing your experiences, any changes you've noticed, and any concerns you have helps the practitioner tailor the treatment to better meet your needs.

Be honest and detailed in your feedback to ensure that the adjustments made are based on accurate information.

Adjusting goals is also important as you progress through treatment. Initially set goals may need modification based on your evolving needs and the improvements you are experiencing.

For example, if you reach a goal sooner than expected or if your priorities change, updating your goals can help keep the treatment aligned with your current needs.

Collaboration with your practitioner to adjust the treatment plan or set new goals ensures that you continue to make progress and address any new issues that may arise.

This dynamic approach to treatment helps in achieving optimal results and maintaining motivation throughout the process.

Maintaining Results: Strategies To Maintain Improvements Over Time

Once you've achieved improvements through Structural Integration, maintaining these results requires ongoing effort. One key strategy is to incorporate exercises and stretches recommended by your practitioner into your daily routine. These exercises help to sustain the benefits gained and prevent regression.

Regular self-care practices, such as maintaining good posture, staying active, and practicing mindfulness, also play a significant role in preserving results.

Developing healthy habits that support your physical well-being can contribute to long-term success.

Additionally, periodic check-ins with your practitioner can be beneficial.

These sessions allow you to review your progress, address any emerging issues, and receive guidance on maintaining the improvements you've achieved.

By staying proactive and engaged, you can effectively sustain the positive changes made during your treatment.

Periodic Reviews: Scheduling Follow-Up Sessions And Reviews

Scheduling periodic reviews is an essential component of maintaining progress and ensuring that treatment continues to be effective.

These follow-up sessions provide an opportunity to evaluate how well you've maintained the improvements and to address any new or ongoing issues.

Typically, follow-up sessions are scheduled at intervals determined by your practitioner, based on your individual needs and progress. During these reviews, your practitioner will assess your current condition, discuss any changes since the last session, and adjust the treatment plan if necessary.

It's important to attend these reviews regularly, as they help in monitoring long-term progress and in making timely adjustments to the treatment plan.

Consistent follow-up ensures that you continue to benefit from the treatment and that any potential setbacks are addressed promptly.

Self-Assessment: Tools For Self-Assessment And Reflection

Self-assessment is a valuable tool for monitoring your progress and reflecting on the effectiveness of the treatment. Various tools and techniques can aid in this process, such as self-assessment questionnaires, mood and pain logs, and personal reflection journals.

Self-assessment questionnaires often include questions about your current pain levels, functional abilities, and overall well-being.

By regularly completing these questionnaires, you can track changes over time and identify patterns that might indicate improvements or areas needing attention.

Maintaining a reflection journal where you record your experiences, feelings, and any observations about your body's response to treatment can also provide insights.

This personal documentation helps in understanding how the treatment is impacting your daily life and in making informed decisions about any necessary adjustments.

Using these self-assessment tools alongside professional evaluations ensures a comprehensive approach to monitoring progress and maintaining the benefits of Structural Integration.

CHAPTER NINE

COMMON CONCERNS AND FAQS

Safety And Risks: Addressing Common Safety Concerns And Risks

Structural Integration is generally considered safe, but like any therapeutic practice, it's important to be aware of potential risks. A key concern is that some people might experience discomfort or soreness after sessions, similar to how muscles might feel sore after a workout. This is usually temporary and should resolve within a few days. It's crucial to communicate openly with your practitioner about any discomfort you're experiencing, as they can adjust their approach to better suit your needs.

Another safety consideration involves ensuring that your practitioner is well-trained and certified. Structural Integration practitioners should have thorough training in anatomy, physiology, and the techniques of the practice. Before starting sessions, check their credentials and ask about their experience. If you have any medical conditions or injuries, inform your practitioner beforehand to ensure that the treatment is tailored to your specific needs and is safe for you.

Cost And Accessibility: Understanding The Financial Aspects And Accessibility Of Sessions

The cost of Structural Integration can vary depending on the practitioner's location, experience, and the length of the session. On average, sessions range from $100 to $200 per hour, with packages often available for a reduced rate if multiple sessions are booked. While this may seem expensive, many people find the investment worthwhile for the benefits they receive.

Accessibility can also be a concern. Structural Integration practitioners are not available everywhere, and finding one in your area might require some research. You can start by searching online directories or asking for referrals from healthcare professionals. If you live in a location where access to practitioners is limited, consider contacting practitioners who offer remote consultations or searching for nearby cities where services might be more readily available.

Finding A Practitioner: Tips For Finding A Qualified Structural Integration Practitioner

Finding a qualified Structural Integration practitioner involves several steps. Start by looking for practitioners who are certified by reputable organizations such as the Guild for Structural Integration or the International Association of Structural Integration.

These certifications ensure that the practitioner has met specific training and competency standards.

You can also seek recommendations from healthcare professionals or individuals who have experienced Structural Integration.

Online reviews and testimonials can provide insights into a practitioner's effectiveness and approach.

It's important to schedule a consultation before committing to a full series of sessions. This initial meeting allows you to discuss your goals, ask questions, and get a sense of the practitioner's style and how comfortable you feel with them.

Session Frequency: How Often You Should Schedule Sessions

The frequency of Structural Integration sessions depends on your individual needs and goals.

For many people, a series of 10 sessions, spaced about one to two weeks apart, is recommended to achieve the best results. This series allows for progressive changes in the body to be integrated effectively over time.

After completing the initial series, the frequency of maintenance sessions can vary. Some individuals choose to schedule follow-up sessions every few months, while others might only return for sessions as needed.

Your practitioner can guide how often you should come in based on your progress and any ongoing issues.

Long-Term Benefits: What To Expect In The Long Run And How To Sustain Benefits

Structural Integration can offer numerous long-term benefits, including improved posture, reduced chronic pain, and enhanced movement efficiency. Many people report a greater sense of physical balance and alignment, which can lead to increased overall well-being and comfort in daily activities.

To sustain the benefits of Structural Integration, it's important to maintain a healthy lifestyle. Regular exercise, good posture practices, and staying hydrated can all contribute to keeping your body in balance. Additionally, periodic follow-up sessions with your practitioner can help address any new issues and maintain the progress you've achieved.

Structural Integration can be a valuable investment in your physical health and well-being. By addressing common concerns and understanding the practical aspects of this practice, you can make informed decisions and enjoy the full range of benefits it offers.

www.ingramcontent.com/pod-product-compliance
Lightning Source LLC
Chambersburg PA
CBHW061301250726
48653CB00002B/729